Childbirth

As told by Childbirth Educator, Melissa Ross

Copyright 2016

Seattle, Washington

Createspace

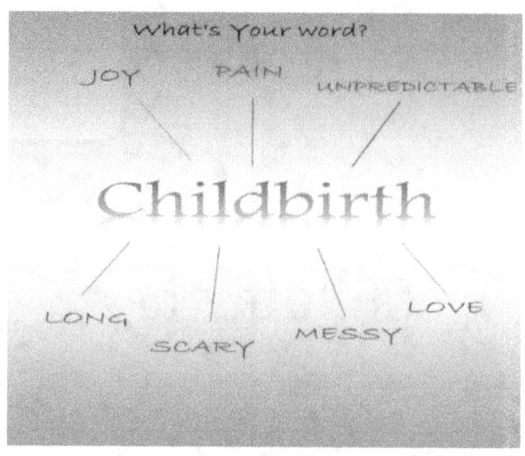

Did you notice the main word missing from this snapshot of what most people think about when they hear the word,
"CHILDBIRTH?"

How about this word, "BABY!"???????

Most people get most of their exposure to child birth from sitcoms and movies, plus through stories from anyone and everyone about their brother's sister's mother's horrible labor. So it is not surprising this leaves us with way more RED (fear-based) words than GREEN (calm) words in relation to birth.

My goal, through creating this book, is to give you lots of information so you have the tools to deal with the RED words and focus on the GREEN words.

Think of me as an afterschool special – *Knowledge is Power!*

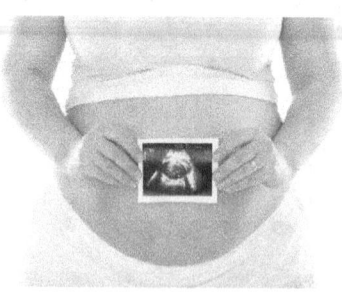

CHILDBIRTH

Congratulations! You're having a baby! So much to look forward to and so much planning and prep.

I'm hoping that you are taking good care of yourself and taking "me time" as much as you can. You will be very busy with a little one soon and you should spoil yourself now.

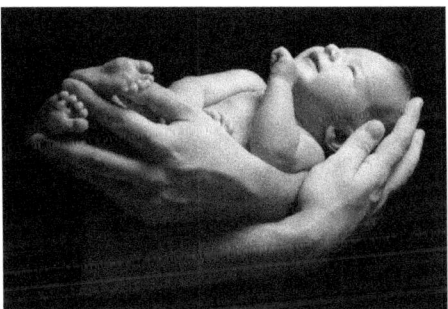

So let's chat about having that baby and getting you ready for not only childbirth but beyond as well. Perhaps you have a partner. Perhaps you have a village of people. Perhaps you have *you*. All of those scenarios can work just fine in these arenas of childbirth and parenting, but I do hope you have some people you trust and can lean on. We want you to stay connected and accept help when it's offered, at least while you are recovering after birth. You are going to be a great mom! You already are! Look at you! Planning ahead, learning all you can to be ready –

WHO AM I?

I am a C.B.E., C.B.D., C.G.E., and A.M.O.F. Impressed yet? I didn't think so. To break it down and endorse the info I am bringing to you in this great little book, I am a Certified Birth Educator, Certified Birth Doula, Certified Gottman Educator and an Amazing Mom of Four. Lots of initials to get the point across that I am a birth junkie that teaches many classes at local hospitals in the Seattle area and has attended many births of wonderful Seattle families, along with lived to tell about the four births of my own. I also am a real estate agent – great dual career combo! Anyway, point is – I am passionate about birth and families and wrote this book to empower moms and families-to-be with lots of great information about hospital births, what to expect and how to be prepared.

And just as a warning, I do tell some corny jokes as we travel along. Groan, roll your eyes, whatever you need to muddle through them because here's the deal – I am saying all the scary words and you then have to read all those words – and sometimes, humor, even the painful kind, can help us feel a little less scared and a little less worried. Laughter has been shown to reduce blood pressure, decrease stress and be a natural pain killer. We all could use more giggles! So here we go-

Please do note that every hospital is different, as are every OBGYN and midwife. My descriptions, as we travel through birth, are general and generic on purpose. They are meant to provide you as much mental prep as possible for your individual labor and delivery.

The book itself is also meant as a spring-board for you to ask lots of questions of the experts around you, as you travel through pregnancy, giving you even more knowledge on what to expect. I am not an OBGYN or a midwife, but an educator.

Your birth will be an original – perfectly unlike anyone else's before or after – and a story you will share hundreds of times. Believe in yourself and your strength – advocate for yourself – ask for help if you need or want it – and try to enjoy this magical event – It's truly life-changing!

LABOR AND BIRTH

- Discomforts in the Third Trimester (or sooner)
- Warnings Signs
- Pre-Term Labor
- Contractions – Purpose / Types
- Am I in Labor????
- Phases and Stages of Labor
  - Early Labor
  - Active Labor
  - Transition
  - Pushing and Delivery
  - Placenta Delivery

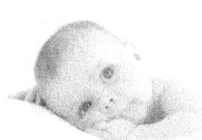

- Breathing Techniques for Labor
- Coping Techniques for Labor
- Birth Plans
- Doulas
- General Hospital Procedures
- Monitoring – External / Internal
- Pain Medications
- Induction
- Augmentation
- Second Stage Interventions
- C-Sections

Aches and pains during pregnancy are normal and expected, especially in the final trimester, as baby gets bigger and organs are losing real estate in your body. Below is a great reference chart on the most common and expected discomforts, along with their cause (other than the fact you are growing a human) and how they might be alleviated. Note that many are tied to your hydration, so before you get cozy to read this section, fill your water bottle and take some sips while you check out the chart.

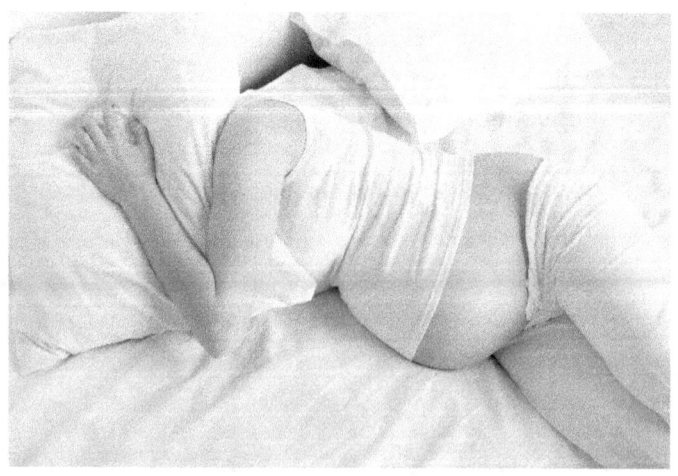

DISCOMFORT	CAUSE	SOLUTIONS
Varicose Veins	Increased pressure of the baby on lower body, which restricts blood flow and causes it to pool in veins.	Elevate legs as often as possible and with pillows while sleeping. Reduce standing times. Avoid nylons, choose compression socks instead.
Hemorrhoids	Constipation Increased pressure on rectum and perineum, cause slower blood flow.	Soak in warm bath. Shift weight off your bottom. Apply ice pack, witch hazel or hemorrhoid cream to rectum for relief.
Constipation	Compression of rectum by uterus. Pregnancy hormones slow process of waste removal.	Walks and light exercise. Water (8+ glasses/day) and prune juice. High-fiber grains, raw vegetables and fruit, beans. Daily stool softener.
Backache	Strain from pregnancy weight gain. Ab muscles stretched and weakened.	Warm/cold compresses. Sleep on your side/firm mattress/pillow between legs Good posture and back stretches/exercises.
Leg Cramps	Increased pressure on nerves leading to legs. Decreased blood circulation.	Massage of legs. Walking and exercise. Straighten leg

		and flex foot toward you to relieve cramps.
Insomnia	Freq. urination. Night sweats / anxiety. Discomfort/active baby.	Avoid late in day caffeine. Warm bath before bed. Body pillow for sleeping.
Heartburn	Growing uterus pushes up on stomach, which can allow stomach acid to leak into esophagus.	Avoid food right before bed. Try 6 small meals instead of 3 big meals and avoiding greasy/spicy/acidic foods. Prop upper body up with pillows at bedtime. Hydration, hydration.

I'm hoping you are under the care of a healthcare practitioner and you feel safe and comfortable with them and their level of care. I also hope that they have covered these warning signs – things to notice – and call them if you experience one or more of them. You can call your healthcare practitioner as often as you need, although not listed as a perk in their flyers, because especially first time moms-to-be, have a lot of questions and a lot of worries. Don't hesitate to reach out to them. You should also be able to call the hospital that you are delivering at and speak to a nurse in Labor and Delivery or Labor Triage, if you cannot get through to your OB or Midwife, or if you worry you have called too many times *today*.

Call your healthcare provider if you have one or more of these symptoms:

- Swelling – normal to have some in your ankles and feet but if not alleviated with putting feet up/sleep and ample hydration, or if you have sudden or overnight swelling in face and hands, could be symptoms of bigger problem and tied to blood pressure.
- Major change in baby's movement
- Vision problems or headache – try to drink big glass of water first – if no relief, call in.
- Pain or burning with urination that continues
- Vaginal bleeding not tied to a vaginal exam
- Vomiting or diarrhea that lasts 24 hours or longer
- Sudden pain in belly
- Fever that is above 100 degrees F (37.7 degrees C)

Research has found that the best thing for babies is to continue growing in utero until at least 39 weeks for the best lung growth and development. We also know that your "Due Date" is an estimate, and could be off by a week or so. So basically, more often than not, longer in utero is better for baby. Preterm labor is labor that begins prior to the 37th week mark of pregnancy. Paying close attention to what is happening with your body is very important throughout pregnancy, especially the last trimester. If you are experiencing one or more of the symptoms listed below, it is important to call your health provider or delivery hospital right away.

Preterm Labor Signs

- Lower belly or pelvic pressure that isn't going away.
- Your water breaks in a gush or a trickle.
- Change/increase in vaginal discharge (bloody, watery or mucus-like)
- Dull ache in pelvic area, lower back, lower belly and or upper thighs
- Mild cramps in belly area (with or without diarrhea)
- Regular or frequent contractions that show a pattern of 4 or more in an hour (may not have pain, just tightening)

You've heard the word but what the heck are they? Labor contractions are the tightening and relaxing of the uterine muscle, which is the largest muscle in a woman's body. The tightening begins at the top of the uterus and then radiates down. Contractions have two jobs – to efface and dilate the cervix – or to thin out and open up the cervix. There are three types of contractions. Let's break them down-

- **Braxton Hicks Contractions** – these can begin as early as 20 weeks and often do not have pain associated with them. They are basically your uterine muscle practicing for the big event, but they have no pattern and truthfully, many first time moms don't even realize they are having them. They often feel like a tightening of the belly that lasts about 20-30 seconds and then relaxes. But because with first pregnancies, everything is still very tight, you may not notice them. Don't worry, your uterus will still be ready when it's time!

- **Mild Contractions** – these are the starters and begin very low on the radar. Laboring women can talk and walk through these, and hopefully sleep through many of them as well. They may begin to feel similar to menstrual cramps, somewhat achy and more noticeable.

- **Non-Mild Contractions** (*try not to use many scary words in this book*) – these are the big ones and pretty hard to sleep through these. Laboring women will have a hard time walking or talking through these and will need to be supported while coping with this type of contraction. These are necessary to do the big work of labor.

One of the very first jobs for your support person will be to time these mild contractions. You or they will need to know the answer to these two questions every time you call in to your healthcare provider once labor has begun to determine the next step in the process:

1. How long does each contraction last?
2. How far apart are the contractions?

So to time a contraction, you would begin when the belly starts to tighten and continue timing until the belly has completely relaxed.

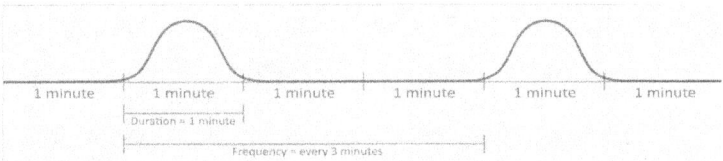

To time how far apart they are, time from the start of one contraction to the start of the next contraction.

Realistically, you will not be using a stop watch, paper and pen. More likely you will be using a contraction timing app on your smart phone. You should go look at the over 25 choices right now on your phone's store platform and download it. No seriously, put the book down and go do it. You don't want to forget and then be trying to find Wi-Fi on the big day and have no idea how it works. Go pick one and play with it for a bit. Create some different scenarios and have some fire drills. You'll be happy you did. *I'll wait right here for you.*

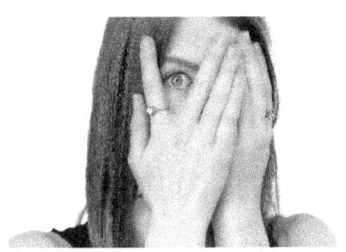

So the very real question that will begin to run on a loop in your mind, especially as you inch closer and closer to your due date – "Am I in labor?" "Am I going to go in to labor tonight?" "Where are you going? I might go in to labor!" – is very intense and I want to give you some tools to know if it really, truly is labor or if it is your body creating a fire drill and possibly false labor.

So let's talk scenario and the tests you can do to see. Say you start to experience contractions and they seem to keep coming.

The first thing you will need to do is:

1. **Drink a big glass of water**

   If the contractions start to subside and then go away, it was your uterus sending up a flare and letting you know that your body is dehydrated. Drink more water!

   If that doesn't stop contractions-

2. **Empty your bladder**

   If the contractions start to subside and then go away, it was your bladder, who knows you are already very annoyed with it, letting you know that you shouldn't be holding your urine and you need to make more frequent trips to the bathroom. That poor bladder has lost most of its real estate and can barely hold anything at this point.

   If these two actions do not stop contractions-

3. **Lay down or at least put your feet up and relax for 30-60 minutes**

If the contractions start to subside and then go away, most likely it was your body letting you know to start working half days or to stop hanging out with people that are stressing you out. Time to take some me-time and slow down. Your body and your baby will thank you.

If you have done all three of these actions, and contractions keep coming, then you are experiencing **Progressive Contractions** and you are most likely in true labor. If it is preterm in your pregnancy (prior to 37 weeks), contractions can sometimes be stopped with medication so that baby can stay a bit longer in utero. It is time to start timing them, looking for a pattern and calling your healthcare provider. Progressive contractions will slowly start to get stronger, longer and closer together. This is one of the two ways you can know that labor has started and you will get to meet your baby soon!

Another way we know that labor has begun is if your **water has broken** – the amniotic sac that is surrounding your baby

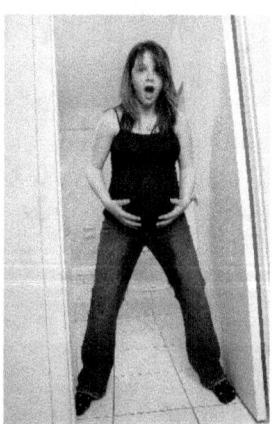

has ruptured. About 10-12% of labors begin this way.

There is no way to stop labor if your water breaks. You will be meeting your baby within the next 36 hours, at the longest.

It can break in two ways – a gush or a trickle.

A *gush* is hard to miss or be in denial about. It is usually about a cup or more of amniotic fluid.

A *trickle* is easier to be in denial about, especially if you haven't finished the nursery or have a meeting to go to. It's also easy to miss because in the last couple weeks of pregnancy, that poor bladder can barely hold a drop, and it is very common to have some urine leaks – so easy to confuse the two. If you sway your hips back and forth and continue to trickle, most likely your water has broken.

Either way, once it breaks, you will first need to call your support person, if they are not with you, and next, you will need to call your healthcare provider.

They will ask you 4 questions to determine the next step in your labor:

> **T** ime – what time did not notice the fluid?
>
> A mount – approximate amount to give them idea of trickle or gush
>
> C olor – should be clear with (maybe) a little pink
>
> O dor – should just smell like mom, maybe body odor smell

Most of the time, when a woman's water breaks, she is told to come in to the healthcare provider's office for a well-check appointment to insure it is truly amniotic fluid and to see how baby is handling this change to their environment. If there are contractions, and there isn't always, they will also time them and check mom's blood pressure. After these assessments, many women are then sent to labor at home for a while. Most hospitals, with low risk pregnancies, want laboring women to make some progress at home, comfortable in their own environment. One of the keys with keeping labor in motion, is relaxation, and being able to be in your own familiar environment, petting your dog, eating your own food, etc., can be one way to achieve some form of relaxation. Sometimes contractions are coupled with your water breaking, sometimes it could take 12 hours for contractions to show up. And sometimes, our uteruses don't start contracting on their own and a medical intervention will need to happen to get them started. We will talk more about that in the medical section.

Variances

1. Occasionally, the amniotic fluid could have color to it – bright red, brown, green, yellow or versions of any of those.

This is very often a sign that baby has had their first bowel movement in utero and that waste is now floating in their environment. This would be reason to go directly to your delivery hospital (per your healthcare provider instructions), where you would, depending on how baby is doing, be either taken directly in for an unplanned C-section to get baby out delivered quickly or be continuously monitored and still be able to have a successful vaginal delivery.

2. Occasionally, the amniotic fluid has a strong odor, which you will notice. This can be a sign of an infection in utero. This variance also means going directly to the hospital (per your healthcare provider instructions), where they can determine the next step. They would most likely do continual monitoring of baby to make sure they are handling this variance and monitoring of mom as well. Sometimes, infections can be treated with medication and monitoring and a vaginal delivery can still be possible. Sometimes though, it also can mean delivery must happen in an unplanned C-section. Many factors would be taken under consideration to determine your specific and individual plan.

Some other signs that labor is coming soon – maybe in two weeks, but still soon are:

- Loss of the mucus plug – this thick plug has kept the uterus sealed during pregnancy and usually comes out when the cervix begins to thin. This can happen weeks before labor or minutes. When it falls out, it may cause clear, pink, brown or even bloody spotting, or you may notice a glob of mucus. Many women do not even notice the loss of it.
- Strong nesting instinct – Urge to alphabetize the spices in your pantry, clean or prepare your home for your baby.
- Diarrhea
- Aches in lower back
- A weight-loss of 1-3 pounds

Do you know how long the average first labor lasts for moms-to-be? 18 hours! Yes, you read that correctly – 18 hours. So first of all, that is not (usually) 18 hours of profanity and pain. Many families get most of their initial exposure to childbirth via sitcoms and movies and although there is a small amount of truth to some of the scenarios you may have seen, most of the material they draw from reality falls in the shortest phase of labor. To get this average of 18 – you need two ends of the spectrum – those being 6 hours to 24 hours. Let's compare it to digging a ditch. I probably need to come up with a better comparison, but let's go with it for now. If you were asked to dig a ditch in 6 hours, with no rest, no breaks, no water or nourishment and no support – that would be pretty tough on your mental and physical state and quite a lot to ask of your body. Alternately, if you dug the same ditch over 24 hours, with many opportunities for rest, nourishment, support, etc. – that would be a lot kinder to your body and your mental state. And truthfully, it can also be kinder to Baby. So let's break down the stages and phases so you know more what to expect.

~~~~~~

EARLY LABOR – longest phase – lasts 6-12 hours for first labors – dilation from 0 – 4 cm

- Mild to moderate phase
- Mild contractions arrive – mom can walk and talk through, maybe sleep through many
- Contractions last 30 – 45 seconds
- Contractions are anywhere from 5 – 30 minutes apart
- Warm up phase of labor
- Lots of potential for rest in this phase
- Circle of awareness is largest, so doesn't need side-by-side support in early part of this phase
- Emotions are *excitement* – "Yay! We're having a baby!"
  - Then *anxiety* – "Oh my gosh, we're having a baby!"

- Partners/Support people – this is the phase that jokes are still funny!
- Important for support people to get to laboring mom, not staying at work or heading into a meeting/sporting event, etc. Emotions and contractions can change suddenly and we want our laboring mom supported and feeling safe.
- This can be a long phase and one our mom will draw a majority of her memories from because she will be most herself in this phase. This time in the labor can be a sweet and positive time – go for a walk together, have some ice cream and cuddle during a Netflix marathon. Enjoy this last phase of being a twosome – before starting your new adventure as a threesome!

Jobs during this phase:

1. Change positions frequently – gravity and movement are your friends in labor – take their help.
2. Drink water – especially after every contraction. Many moms get dehydrated in labor and have to have IV fluids, which means you are attached to an IV. If you get in the habit early, this can make a difference and can help keep labor progressing.
3. Eat! - Small meals are a good idea because there's not much room for your stomach to expand and nausea usually shows up during labor. Stick with foods that will give you as much energy at the end as possible – think about it being a marathon – protein and carbs. Truthfully, if it sounds good – eat it. Even the World Health Organization believes moms should eat throughout labor, as long as they are unmedicated and low risk.
4. Empty your bladder – this one might seem silly – especially if your partner/support person is reminding you to go to the bathroom every hour – but you will become a less willing participant in this activity, so get in the habit early. It is also a way to keep labor progressing.

Soapbox moment – I've been lucky to be present at many, many births and I have also caught a number of dads during labor. Here's why – they did a fantastic job, taking care of mom, giving her ice chips every two minutes, breathing with her during every contraction, slow dancing with her, giving her massages, etc. They probably never left her side. And then, when baby's head begins to crown, things get *very* real in a Labor and Delivery room, and this is often when dads lose their legs and go down. So although they did a fabulous job caring for laboring mom, they did not put food and hydration into their own body and that all catches up to them at the crowning moment. Make sure our support people know that they need to take care of themselves while they are taking care of you – we want them there for the whole show, not sipping orange juice in the corner during the best part of the show!

Getting from EARLY LABOR *to* ACTIVE LABOR – Dilation from 3 – 6 cm

- Moderate to hard phase
- Cervix tends to resist dilation until very thin
- Contractions last 45 – 60 seconds
- Contractions are 3 – 5 minutes apart
- Intense but slow phase of labor
- Emotions and physical changes begin and mom needs lots more support now

Basically, this is one of the most challenging parts of labor and can take a while. ⸙

ACTIVE LABOR – lasts 3 – 5 hours for first time labors – Dilation from 6 – 8

- Hard phase
- Non-mild contractions – these are hard for mom to walk or talk through – may have arrived late in EARLY LABOR as well
- Contractions last 45 – 60 seconds
- Contractions are 2 – 4 minutes apart
- Intensity increases
- Circle of awareness is much smaller – mom needs support during every contraction or her fear and anxiety will be running the show
- Jokes are no longer funny
- This is the phase that you are either at hospital or on your way – using **5.1.1.** to help determine (contractions are 5

minutes apart / they are lasting for 1 minutes / pattern exists for 1 hour)

- Noise – laboring women start to instinctually make noise – moan/groan/mantras – can't plan or predict what will come out of you but it's all normal! *(story below)
- Nausea can show up, along with vomiting
- Can be the most frustrating phase for our laboring families – many labors stall/stop between the dilation of 4cm and 7cm for a variety of reasons – meaning that perhaps at 1 pm you had a vaginal exam during your laboring at the hospital. Your birth team told you that you were dilated to 5cm – Yay! Half way there! But then, they return to do another vaginal exam at 6pm and tell you that you are still only dilated to 5cm. *What?* So not fair! You've been doing everything and coping with non-mild contractions for 5 hours and no progress? What gives? Well, we don't always know what stalls labor – could be stress, could be exhaustion, could be a grouchy uterus (not a medical term) – basically many things could contribute and it's very common. We have medical interventions that can get the show back on the road though. This too, we will talk more about in the medical section.
- Partners/Support People need to take on more of a coaching role during this phase – giving mom lots of support, encouragement and guidance.

Jobs during this phase

1. Change positions frequently – gravity and movement are your friends in labor – take their help.
2. Drink water – especially after every contraction.
3. Eat! – If you are still interested in food, a clear diet may be recommended now. Hospitals usually have nourishment rooms on Labor and Delivery floors that have ample popsicles, jello, juice, crackers and ice.
4. Empty your bladder – Here is where you may begin to not want to participate in this activity and the reason being that you may not want to have a contraction in the bathroom by yourself. Have an honest conversation with your support person about who might be able to go in to the bathroom with you to help you cope with a contraction while trying to go the bathroom.

TRANSITION – shortest phase – 30 minutes – 2 hours – dilation from 8cm – 10cm

- Hardest phase
- Contractions last 60 – 90 seconds
- Contractions are now coming every 1 – 3 minutes
- Intensity increases even more – not because of a pain increase but because of how close the contractions are now coming – similar to being in the ocean and waves keep crashing over your head – hard to catch your breath and little time to rest – laboring women have a hard time communicating in long explanations here – short statements are more common
- Nausea arrives if it hasn't already
- Laboring moms often cry when this phase begins due to intensity / emotions are strong
- This is the phase that sitcoms/movies get their material from due to the details
- "I QUIT!" Can often be heard from a non-medicated laboring mom in transition because she is overwhelmed. Very normal!
- Sensory signals are increased and off the charts so laboring mom is very sensitive to:

    smells – that cologne partner put on before leaving for the hospital now makes mom   want to vomit/ garlic at lunch, perfumed lotion, etc...

    hot/cold – layers of clothing feel restrictive – she may want cold wash cloth and a heating pad

    lights – best to keep them low

    sounds – music may need to go off or different playlist

    people – laboring moms are very overwhelmed during this phase so support people need to be close and giving lots of verbal encouragement and guidance

Jobs during this phase

1. Change positions frequently – if laboring mom still wants to move around

2. Drink water – or ice chips if nausea arrives
3. Empty your bladder – during this phase, the pelvic pressure is intense, and now when it's time to go to the bathroom, it will be difficult to urinate and may feel like baby could fall into the toilet! Don't worry – unless you are two months early in your delivery, this would be pretty difficult to accomplish. It is also very likely you will have contractions in the bathroom, so be sure someone from your support team goes into the restroom with you to provide support and reassurance.

Support people need to give lots of encouragement and emotion support during this phase since mom is very overwhelmed.

PUSHING AND DELIVERY

- Dilation is complete
- Contractions are 60 – 90 seconds long
- Contractions are 3 – 5 minutes apart
- Some women, upon dilating to 10 am, will have an undeniable urge to push. For other laboring moms, that instinct could take up to 20-30 minutes to occur. Most birth teams will wait for that instinct to occur – called Laboring Down – in order to give her uterus, the chance to catch up to baby. If instinct isn't apparent right away, they should be allowing mom to rest until instinct happens – often a light 20-minute nap.
- Bowel movements – this is an area that most expectant moms have some anxiety about when thinking about labor and pushing. You will be using every ounce of energy in your body to push out that little one and yes, bowel movements do occur – quite frequently actually – about 85% of vaginal deliveries. So because it happens so often, the birth teams expect it to happen and no one is running around your Labor and Delivery room

freaking out because of it. Just like the blood, tissue and amniotic fluid that you are also pushing out of your body, they want everything out of the way so that it the safest environment for baby to arrive. Most moms have no idea if they were in the 85% either – *they rarely ask.* The only people who make any fuss over it are partners/support people. So it's a good idea to share this paragraph with them and have an honest conversation with them about any anxiety or worry you may be carrying so that they can be aware and supportive.

- Positions – they are at least 5 different options for pushing and you should keep trying them until you find one you like and clicks for you. If you are medicated with an Epidural, your choices drop to only two, due to being numb in your legs. See options below: (note that each hospital is different on their offerings, so it's good to ask on your tour of your delivery hospital or healthcare provider what options are available for you)

Side-Lying – Available when medicated (Epidural) or un-medicated. When a contraction begins, knee is lifted out and toward chest, pulling knee toward you, while pushing at the same time. If medicated, you may need assistance holding leg. When contraction is over, leg is set down and you go as limp and relaxed as possible.

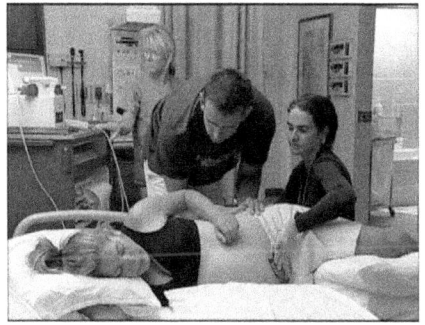

Squatting Bar – In many hospitals, squatting is a great option during pushing because it can open the pelvis up to 30 % more. That can be a little kinder for your body and maybe a little easier for baby's journey. A squatting bar is available in many hospitals, being added to the end of your bed. You could lean over the bar,

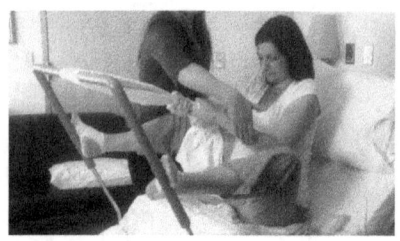 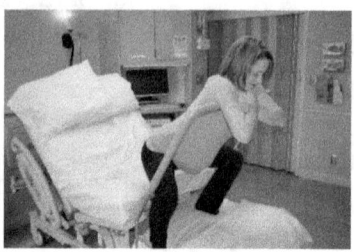

using it support some of your weight – or you could wrap a sheet or towel around the bar, brace your feet on the legs of the bar, and pull back. Both of these could be options ONLY if you do not have an epidural since you would not have control of your legs and be unable to support yourself safely.

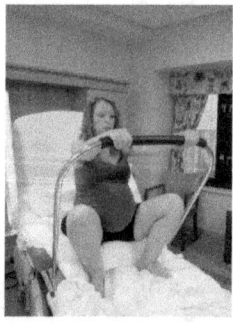

Squatting Forward – Here is another great squatting option available if you are *not* using an Epidural. With this position, you would be leaning toward your bed, either into the head of your bed or wrapped around pillows on your bed, with your legs in a squatting position. Many babies are actually *delivered* in this position!

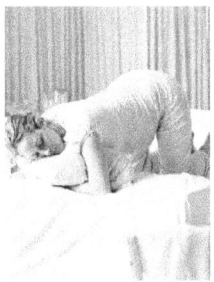 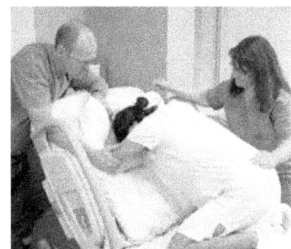

Birth Stool – This is another unmedicated option for our laboring moms that is available in many hospitals. A Birth Stool can be a great option for a mom that is struggling with pushing and really having a hard time getting the concept of it or able to do it effectively. By sitting on a Birth Stool, our laboring mom is mimicking a position she does every day with a bowel movement, so may be more successful with the familiarity of it and able to relax enough to make progress.

Usually, by crowning, your healthcare provider would move laboring mom into one of the previously mentioned positions so that they could more efficiently access the vaginal opening to assist with the delivery of baby. The stool does have a hole in it though, along with a sanitized catch basin, if things move quickly or mom prefers stool to the bed.

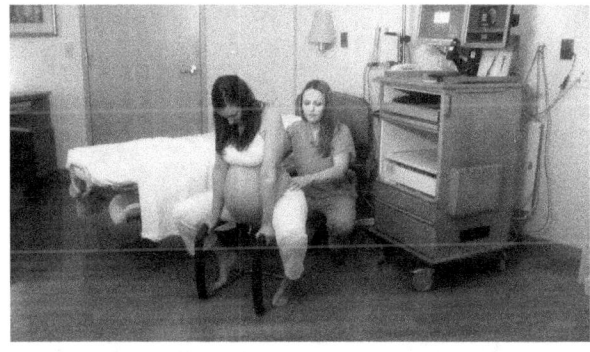

On your back – This option works whether you are unmedicated or medicated and relies on your support person(s) helping to bring one or both of your knees toward your chest during a contraction, with you holding on to your knees, thighs, calves or balls of your feet and pulling them toward your chest while pushing.

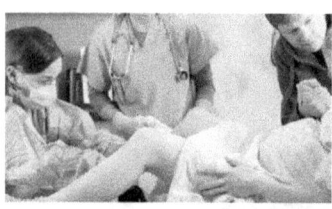 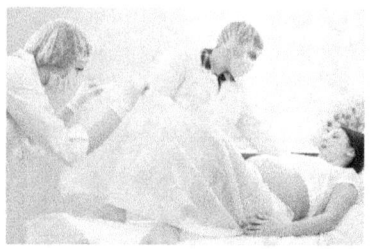

In whatever position you are pushing in, this is basically what you will be doing –

1. When a contraction begins, you will get in to position.
2. Grab a big breath
3. Tuck your chin to your chest
4. Slowly let breathe out while push, push, pushing
5. Grab another big breath
6. Tuck your chin to your chest
7. Slowly let breathe out while push, push, pushing
8. Grab one last big breath
9. Tuck your chin to your chest
10. Slowly let breathe out while push, push, pushing
11. Take a drink or two of water / or ice chips
12. Relax every muscle in your body while you wait for next contraction

It will be very important to rest and relax in between contractions because it is a great deal of work to get baby across that finish line. Partners and support people should also be resting in between contractions.

- Pushing is a 2-step forward / 1-step back process – with Baby making a little progress and then slipping back a bit. This will continue until crowning.
- Crowning – when a baby's head is crowning, this translates to a burning sensation for mom – often referred to as, "The

Burning Ring of Fire." (No relation to Johnny Cash music hit). The reason for this is basically, there is a human trying to exit your body that is larger than the exit. This will cause the skin to stretch, and the pain is translated to burning. When crowning begins, and even beforehand, healthcare providers will start to utilize mineral oil and perineal massage to soften the skin and aide in the exit. They will help ease baby's head out of the vaginal opening, slowly as possible. Then they will help as one shoulder and then the other shoulder is born. Then the rest of baby slips out and they are born! (And that burning sensation goes away!)

Did you notice I did not put the expected time frame on this stage of labor? I did that on purpose because the numbers can be shocking and I wanted to get you through the initial delivery before I told you. Ready? Here goes – pushing for first time labors can take anywhere from 30 minutes to 4 hours or more. Ack! I know! I know! You didn't realize that. Well, fact is – you're in it now – can't get out of this whole labor and delivery so let's talk about those numbers. That birth canal can be a tough one for our little ones to navigate and with the whole slipping back after some progress aspect isn't helping either. It also can take a while to not only find a pushing position you feel comfortable in, but also to just figure out the whole pushing concept in itself. It takes a while for those pushes to actually be making any progress. You'll probably be pretty tired when this stage begins too, so sometimes we have barely any energy left to have effective pushes. Sometimes having a little juice or a popsicle can give you a little boost, if allowed. And truth is, the length of time we now let laboring moms push has increased substantially over the past couple years. Oh yay, you say, right? It really is, "Yay!" though, because the difference in recovering from an additional hour of pushing and recovering from a C-Section because we were only allowed to push for two hours – very different. And all across the country, OBGYNs and Midwives, along with the World Health Organization, are doing lots of proactive things to avoid unnecessary C-Sections when possible. Pushing for a longer period, as long as mom and baby are handling it, is one of those things.

Let's get back to the good stuff – a baby was just born!

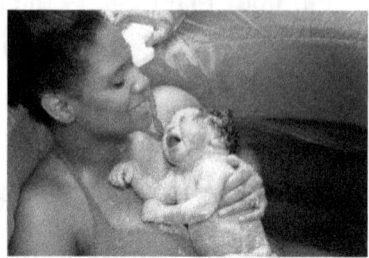

Now what?

Usually, right after baby is born from a vaginal delivery, baby is immediately set on mom's lower abdomen or chest. It is normal for baby to be covered in labor fluids – blood, tissue and amniotic fluid. Baby may also have their first bowel movement on their way out and they may have streaks or meconium as well. Babies also will have vernix on their skin, which looks similar to cream cheese. This has been a wetness barrier on baby while sitting in fluids for the past 9 months and is good for their skin.

Babies can be a bit purplish upon delivery due to an immature circulation system. It usually takes up to 5 minutes for them to pink up. Your delivery team will be monitoring that, along with many other signs of transition for baby. Your birth team will wipe baby's face and use a bulb syringe to remove any labor fluids baby may have taken in through the birth canal and delivery. They will also be rubbing baby all over, to assist that circulation system and warm baby up – it's not about cleaning baby off. Letting the majority of labor fluids and vernix absorb into baby's skin helps to keep their instincts heightened for breastfeeding, so better to wait for baby's first bath as well. In the hospital where I teach, first bathes don't happen for at least 8 – 12 hours after birth. Be sure to ask what your delivery hospital's policy on this is – it's important!

Umbilical Cord

Standard of practice in most labor and delivery hospitals is to leave the umbilical cord attached to baby after delivery for at least 1 minute to 1.5 minutes. When cut at this point, there is still some blood left in the cord so if you are choosing to donate that blood or privately bank it, there is enough to collect. Cord blood is used for stem cell research, as well as in the fight against many diseases like Lymphoma and Leukemia. Good to ask your healthcare provider for additional information on this topic. Another option is to opt for delayed cord clamping, which more and more hospitals and healthcare providers are encouraging and supporting. This basically means leaving the umbilical cord attached to baby until it has brought every last drop of blood and nutrient from the placenta to baby. This process can take anywhere from 3 – 4.5 minutes. If you opt for this process, there will be no blood left in the cord for donation or banking – so one route or the other. The thinking behind the benefits of cord clamping are that this may be the best for baby, giving them extra iron from the extra blood could give them a boost in development and transition. Other schools of thought worry that it could increase their chances of Jaundice. It is very important to have a good and trusting relationship with your healthcare provider so you can speak with them about decisions that need to be made during and after delivery and talk honestly about the pros and cons before making your decisions.

Whenever the cord is going to be cut, in almost every birth, the birth team will ask if partner, support person or even sometimes mom, would like to cut the cord. There are rarer situations, where the cord may need to be cut immediately and by the healthcare provider for the safety of mom and/or baby, as well. If your partner (or yourself) are thinking about cutting the umbilical cord, it's always good to know what to expect.

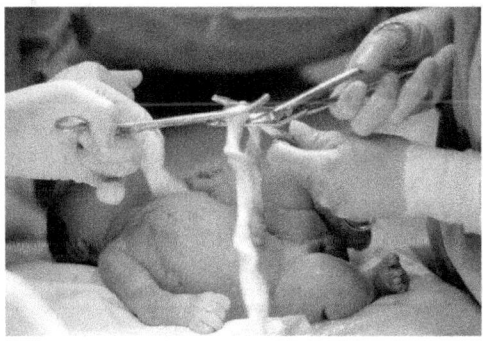

In the picture, you can see a picture of an umbilical cord. You also can see that is surprisingly thick, which means it is not a simple snip, more of a sawing method through rope. Also good to know that there are no nerve endings in the cord, so no one feels the cut. This is also a decision that can be made on the spot, so if you change your mind, no worries.

Once the cord is cut, an adorable hat is put on baby's cone head and they are wrapped in warming blankets and usually brought right up to mom's chest for skin-to-skin time. (Check with your healthcare provider/delivery hospital on their skin-to-skin policies to be sure). Baby will have a cone head for anywhere from 4-6 days after delivery due to the 5 plates in their skull adapting and shifting to travel through the birth canal. Pretty amazing, right? Your photos of baby on day 1 of life will look very different than day 5 of life. Back to skin-to-skin – the blankets will be pulled away from baby's chest and clothing pulled out of the way on mom's chest to make this happen. Skin-to-skin is important for baby's transition to the outside world in many different ways – temperature, breathing, blood sugar, blood pressure, enhances bonding and can help with mom's mood balance due to it promoting production of oxytocin in mom – a hormone that boosts maternal feelings and positive mood. Once baby is placed skin-to-skin with mom, this is usually the moment a tidal wave emotion hits you and your partner or support people. It is wonderful and over-whelming and awesome! Your baby will be fascinated with your voices and faces, as they have been listening to you for the last 9 months and finally get to see you too. Baby's do not always cry right as they are born, but do usually cry within the first 5 minutes of life – which is important so the delivery team can be sure that their lungs are clear and do not have labor fluids impeding breathing. This initial skin-to-skin time is also a great distraction since there is still an audience in your lower region and still some work to be done.

Placenta

It will take your uterus anywhere from 5 – 20 minutes to then deliver your placenta. In that time frame is also when any repairs are done, if needed. It is very common for mom to have a little tearing with a vaginal delivery and a couple dissolvable stitches is usually all that is needed for repair. Many healthcare professionals have moved away from doing episiotomies anymore to open the vaginal opening to accommodate delivery because it is often more likely to have an infection or harder recovery from the surgical cut of an episiotomy than a jagged tear repair. Okay, that's the last time I'll say that word now – no more cringes.

In delivery of your placenta, while holding baby, you will be asked for one or two more good pushes. These are not difficult or even painful – more annoying as you will would rather just focus on your baby. Once your placenta is born, most healthcare providers will try to show you the placenta and I put a picture below. It is pretty amazing that the female body can grow an organ just to grow a baby, shed it and grow it again and again. Spoiler – it is not as cute as your baby. Some families have plans for their placenta – spiritual, cultural, health – if you do, this is something that as to be arranged ahead of time with your healthcare provider and hospital policies do surround it. Ask those questions and make those arrangements *before* labor in order to make that happen for you, if it is something you are planning on.

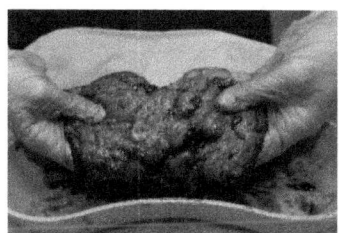

Once your placenta is delivered and repairs are done, the show is over. Your bed is put back together, linen is changed and cleaned up and your birth team starts to be reduced. This is usually a great time for any of your family and friends that may have been pacing the hallways or waiting room, to come in for a quick visit and picture.

*Try to keep visits short initially right after birth, because mom and baby need to start breastfeeding very soon after placenta delivery, and we need mom calm and relaxed for this as well. Too many guests/visitors, can add extra stress on our already nervous and exhausted mom. *

Breastfeeding will be encouraged and taught in the delivery room within the hour after birth. This first hour is called, **"The Golden Hour,"** and is the best time for baby to learn how to breastfeed.

Their instincts are at their peak in this time frame and if we miss getting baby attached to a breast during this window, there is a higher chance that there could be struggles with breastfeeding. Initially, your Labor and Delivery nurses will be assisting you with how to breastfeed, positions and what a good latch looks like and feels like. You will most likely breastfeed baby on both breasts and then baby (and you) will take a nice long nap! You deserve it! Most families are moved to a Postpartum and Recovery Room a couple hours after delivery for the remainder of your stay in the hospital – usually 24 – 36 hours after delivery.

Partners – A good idea for partner to stay in the room, especially the first time learning, so they too can hear directions and see, from a different angle than mom, how to breastfeed. This also shows some of the first signs of support, which can lead to a 50% higher success rate for mom and baby to breastfeed. This can also help mom relax somewhat since ALL moms are nervous about breastfeeding.

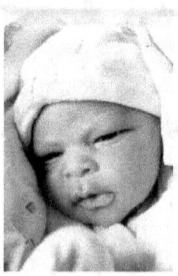

COPING TECHNIQUES

So that was a lot, right? Ready for some techniques to help you with contractions and labor? More than I know, right? Below, I will show you some different positions to try during contractions both at home and at the hospital. Your birth team should also be very familiar with them as well and may have even more ideas to help. Sometimes, encouraging your partner or support person to snap a photo of each of the positions can come in handy and be used as a quick reference once you are in labor. Or, of course, you can take this book with you to your labor and delivery!

BIRTH DOULA

A Birth Doula can be a great addition to your birth team, that can help with support prior to labor, as well as provide comfort techniques, information and guidance during a birth. Some hospitals have them on staff and most welcome them in labor and delivery. They come to your home, if you want, and to the entirety of your labor at the hospital. They assist your partner with coping techniques and empower both of you throughout your special event.

BREATHING

First, let me say, there is no magic breath that will take the pain completely away from a contraction. When you use breathing techniques during labor, it can help create focus during a contraction, reducing room for fear and anxiety, which can reduce some of the pain. When a mom is unfocused or feeling out of control during a contraction, she will often have eyes that are darting around the room and be breathing shallow. And when unfocused, she will be much more uncomfortable because she will be also coping with fear and anxiety. Partners and support people should note the warning signs of an unfocused mom so they know when to step in, take control and help her get back in control. Breathing can be one way to achieve that.

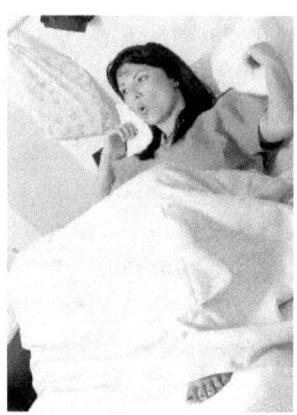

Deep Cleansing Breath – If you practice yoga or meditation, you are probably very familiar with deep cleansing breaths. This type of breath can be a great way to *start* and *end* a contraction. What it is, is a big breath in through your nose and then releasing that breath slowly through your mouth. Did you try it? You can almost feel your muscles relax a bit when you do these. Try one. Big inhale in through your nose, then slowly exhale through your mouth. Nice! These are a great longer shelf life relaxation tool – I use them daily with a teenage daughter at home. Keep this one in your parenting toolkit!

So what about in between those deep cleansing breaths? – Well, this part often needs to come a bit organically, when you are in the moment so it feels good for mom, but here's some suggestions to try.

1. After initial cleansing breath, close your eyes, breathe as normal pace and try to relax as many muscles as possible during the contraction. As the contraction comes to an end, do another deep cleansing breath to let that contraction go.
2. After starting with a deep cleansing breath, you and partner look at each other and you both try to breathe at a regular

pace, taking comfort in the support of each other. End the contraction with a deep cleansing breath.

3. After first cleansing breathe, partner take coaching role and lay one of his palms flat, the other hand perpendicular in mom's vision, and create a tapping pattern – "Okay honey, look at my hand, 1, 2 3, 4, 5, - breathe – 1, 2, 3, 4, 5 – breathe…." Then as the contraction comes to an end, one more deep cleansing breath to finish it and let it go.

The whole point is to keep mom focused and in control during a contraction, so whether she has her eyes closed, looking at the floor, an ultrasound or baby or watching a support person's tapping hand, focus is the goal. Deep cleansing breaths can also be wonderful communication tools to those around you, that you are having a contraction, and now is not the time to ask mom a bunch of questions, but instead be quiet or help in the support of our laboring mom.

The 3 R's

RELAXATION – One of the keys to keeping a labor progressing and feeling in control of labor is relaxation. You may have some tricks you do now to reduce stress or calm yourself down – all of those could be used. If it is safe for mom and baby – give it a try. (I.E. – Do you go for a walk? Sing loud in the car? Binge watch Scandal? – all up to try!)

Other ideas for relaxation – Breathing techniques (mentioned prior), hydrotherapy (shower or bath can help muscles relax), heating pad or ice on lower back and thighs.

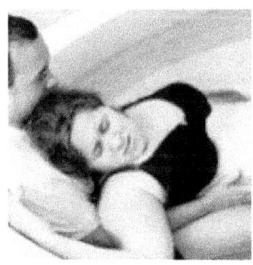

RYTHMN – Swaying your hips from side to side will be a natural instinct behavior that begins in labor as one way your body is coping with labor. This rocking and swaying can ease some of the strain during contractions and feel good to some laboring moms. Music and any type of dancing/movement can also be a great coping technique and a way to keep changing positions and allow gravity to do some of the work of getting baby out. I highly suggest checking out the YouTube videos featuring moms dancing those babies out! Inspiration!

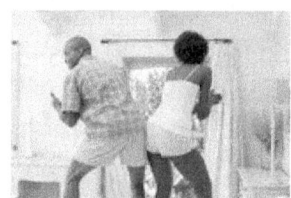

RITUAL – This can provide some comfort to our laboring moms in many ways. Ritual could come from meditation or be prayer-based. Some moms like a script read to them while they are in labor to calm and even focus them. Ritual can also come from unconventional sources. I had a client coping with non-mild contractions and we were still at her home, not time to go to the hospital yet. After one intense contraction, she decided she wanted to vacuum in her living room. One important note to partners and support people, if mom asks to do something while in labor, and it's safe for her and the baby – MAKE IT HAPPEN! So we got her the vacuum and when she wasn't having a contraction, she went around and around the room, vacuuming. When a contraction came, she stopped the vacuum (but did not turn it off), held on to the handle with one hand and leaned against the couch or one of us and rocked and moaned while the contraction happened.

Then as it faded, she went back to vacuuming. The vacuum stayed on for 2.5 hours and she continued her ritual the entire time until it was time to go the hospital. We sadly could not bring the vacuum, but at her home, for that time frame, running the vacuum helped her in a couple ways – 1. The lines created by the vacuum in the carpet, gave her comfort and ritual. 2. The vibration of the vacuum felt calming to her during the contractions and she focused on it, instead of the contraction.

So for her – this worked! She admitted that she never could have predicted she would *want* to vacuum during labor – so be ready for anything.

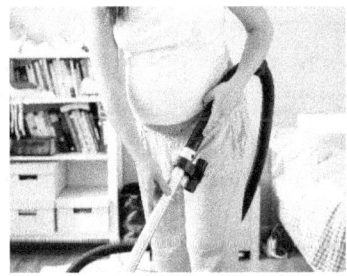

This unconventional example is a great peek at the unpredictability of what might feel right or good to us during labor and that everything is normal. If you find something that is working to keep you calm and in control, keep doing it through your contractions until it is no longer feeling good. You can't predict what your labor will look like, but having a tool bag full of options for comfort is the best way to be ready for anything!

Labor Coping Positions

So as we go through the different positions, note that you can do these at home, outside, at the hospital or pretty much anywhere you feel comfortable.

WALK, WALK, WALK and PAUSE

As long as there is not a medical need to be in bed, we want you to change positions frequently to help baby move through the birth canal. One of the simple ways to do that is to walk – walk around the block, walk down and up the stairs, walk your hospital labor and delivery hallways. But when a contraction comes, it will stop you in your tracks and you will need to cope through it. One way is to lean into the wall, railing, support person, while it's happening. You could also pause and rock back and forth during the contraction.

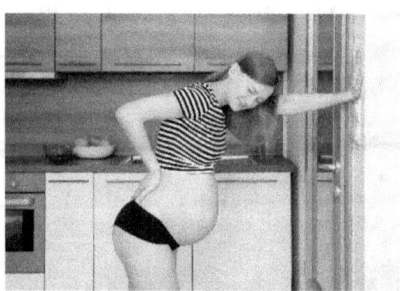
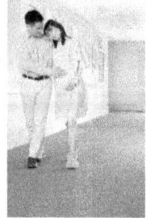

SQUATTING

During labor and pushing, squatting can open up the pelvic area by up to 30% - much nicer to your body. And some laboring moms are drawn to this position. Be sure to give those leg muscles breaks from this position between contractions so legs don't cramp and blood circulation is encouraged. Walking or sitting down in between contractions can achieve this.

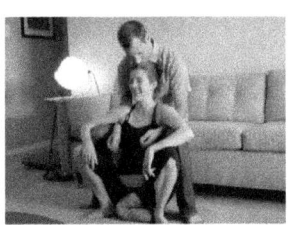 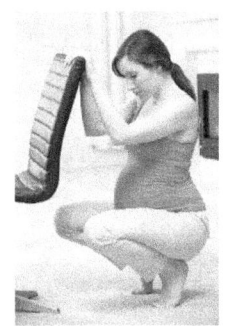

BIRTH BALL (EXERCISE BALL)

A great tool for the last few weeks of pregnancy as it can often be more comfortable to sit on and kinder to your pelvic floor. During labor, it can be used in a variety of ways, as shown below, and also another sitting option for partners and support people in labor and delivery suites. After baby is home, you can also lightly bounce a fussy baby in your arms while gently bouncing on an exercise ball.

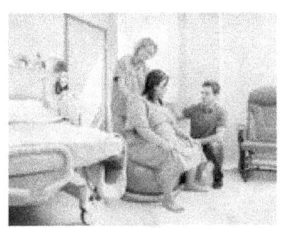 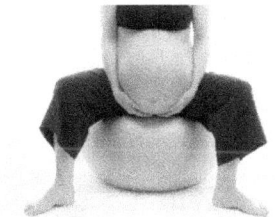

A great longer shelf item comfort tool.

LUNGE

Putting your foot up on a stool or stable chair during a contraction can also be a comfortable way to cope with a contraction, swaying back and forth, leaning into wall or back into a support person. This can also be achieved standing on a staircase and holding onto the railing during a contraction. Be sure to rotate legs when you can and give the leg a break from elevation occasionally as well. Sitting down or walking in between contractions can achieve this so muscles don't cramp and blood continues to circulate well.

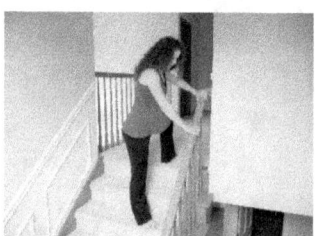

SLOW DANCE

We encourage lots of walking during labor – remember, gravity and movement are your friends – but when a non-mild contraction arrives, it is difficult to continue walking. One option is to slow dance with your partner or support person during the contraction. Lean some of your weight on them and sway/rock your hips back and forth while the contraction tightens, peaks and then relaxes, breathing your way through it.

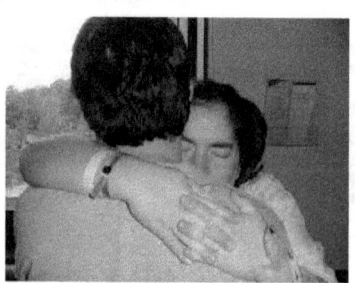

DOWN ON ALL FOURS/FORWARD-LEANING

Some laboring moms are instinctually drawn to this type of coping position because it just *feels* right. These are also both good options if we are still trying to get baby into a more ideal delivery position. Hanging your belly, again using gravity in your favor, can provide just a tiny bit more space for baby to turn. Many partners and support people are unsure how to support mom in these positions though, other than laying on the floor next to them. First of all – don't do that – she won't be a fan. One way a partner could support mom is to use a tennis ball and rub it back and forth on her lower back.

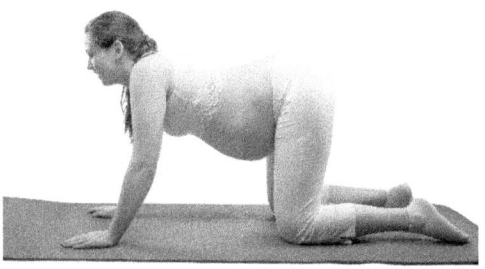

It will hit on many tender pressure points and can feel good to her. You can also roll the tennis ball up and down her back and on her shoulders, easing some of the tension that inevitably builds back there during labor. If you don't have a tennis ball, you can also use a mini hand massager. Hospitals don't usually have these available, so be sure to also have one in your hospital bag.

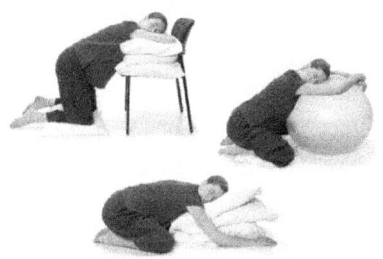

KNEE COMPRESSION

This is a two-fer comfort technique – for expectant moms with lots of lower back aches during pregnancy, this can give you a bit of relief. By pushing on her knees, it opens up the pelvis just a bit, taking some pressure off her lower back and spine area. (Partners also enjoy this after mom-to-be is no longer expecting). It also can be a comfort technique during labor if mom is experiencing back labor – so this would be done *during* a contraction to relieve some of the pressure on her lower back. To do this coping technique, mom sits in a standard size chair that allows her feet to sit flat on the ground. Mom should sit back against the chair and relax, knees together. Support person kneels in front of mom and cups their hands around her knee caps and pushes firmly straight back and holds. No pulsing or lifting of knees, just a steady, firm hold.

DOUBLE HIP SQUEEZE

This is another two-fer comfort technique – again, for expectant moms with lots of lower back aches during pregnancy, this can give her some relief NOW. You would turn this technique into a massage of sorts, especially before bed, helping to relieve some of the soreness and hopefully allow a better sleep. During a contraction, partner / support person would instead hold the squeeze as long as they could to help take some of the pressure off of her lower back and spine.

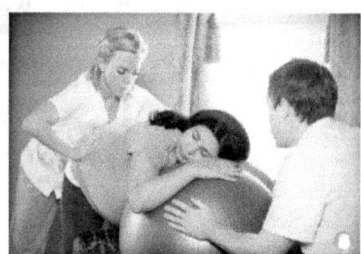

With expectant mom leaning forward in a standing or kneeling position, support person should turn palms in on mom's outer hips and squeeze in and tilt them a bit forward. This should feel good for mom and take a bit of pressure off.

Play with position until you find the right one!

This is often the go-to comfort technique used in labors that have primarily back labor. You can also put your hands together (one on top of the other), and push down on mom's lower back. This is another one mom's in their third trimester really appreciate!

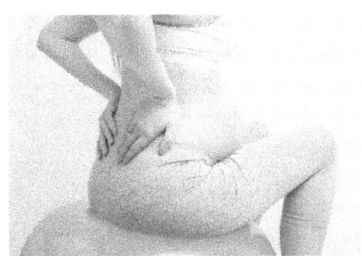
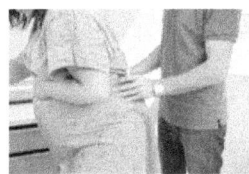

Why would I have back labor? – Most of the time, the reason for back labor is baby's position. The ideal position for baby to be vaginally delivered is anterior – facing mom's back on their way out. Some babies are instead in a posterior position during a vaginal delivery – sometimes called, "Sunny side up,".

When this happens, expectant mom's contractions are primarily in her back and radiate down her legs. You guessed it – not fun. But just because you have back aches during pregnancy – this does not mean baby is in a posterior position – it's because you are growing a human and your body is achy and tired from all it's hard work! Be sure to try the knee compression and double hip squeeze comfort techniques to help with aches and pains *now*. They are not just for labor!

HAND MASSAGE

This a great option for a laboring mom that may not want to be touched a bunch, especially during the Transition Phase, when her sensory signals are really heightened. You can try some of these little massages to stay connected in a small, but still important way.

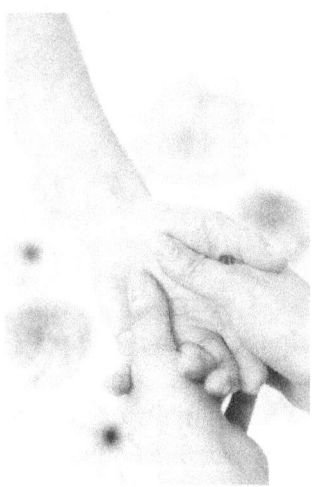

We carry a great deal of tension and stress in our hands, especially in the meaty pad under our thumbs. By massaging the pressure points in our hands, we can help to relieve some of that tension and may be able to relax mom a bit.

Remember – if a laboring mom wants to do something during a contraction, and it's safe for mom and safe for baby, let her do it – make it happen. We want mom to feel in control during contractions so there is less room for anxiety and fear, which means less pain for mom.

I suggest partners/ support people write the following acronym on a bright notecard, fold it up, and put it in their wallet or bag. It will be a helpful reminder of ways to help take care of a laboring mom-

S ET UP OF ENVIRONMENT / SAFE (MUSIC, PEOPLE, SMELLS, TEMP)

U NLOAD BLADDER

P RAISE AND ENCOURAGEMENT

P OSITION CHANGES FREQUENTLY

O UT OF BED AS MUCH AS POSSIBLE

R ELAXATION AND REST

T OUCH AND MASSAGE

Let's walk through what to expect upon arrival to your delivery hospital – in general. Here too, every hospital is different and has differing standards of practice and protocol. I highly recommend you tour your delivery hospital so you can familiarize yourself with not only what the labor and delivery suites look like in advance, but also to find out what their practices and protocol are for labor and delivery. This can help shape your expectations and decisions.

ADMISSION

Once it has been decided that it's time to admit you to the hospital, you can expect to have a few things happen so your birth team can get all the pieces to the puzzle of your labor to help determine the next step. You can expect to fill out some paperwork, even if you have pre-registered. You will also have your temperature taken, your blood pressure assessed and some external monitors put on your belly. (See photo below)

External monitors are basically stretchy belts with transducers that clip on – one belt sits at the top of your belly, one at the lower. The top transducer is paying attention to your contractions – how long they last and how far apart they are. The bottom transducer is paying attention to baby's heartbeat. This is the external way they are seeing how baby is handling labor and contractions. The heartbeat is usually played aloud, which is often quite comforting for expectant parents to hear that familiar noise of their little one. These belts are usually left on for a good 20 minutes to get a good, solid view of how labor is progressing for all parties involved. They

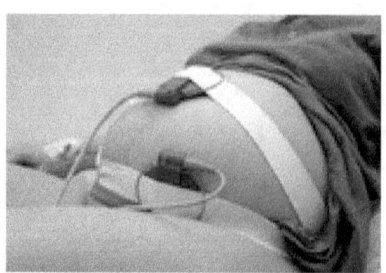

will usually want to monitor you and baby once an hour, for less time than initially, and often have portable and waterproof units available so you don't necessarily have to get in to bed and be tethered to a Machine. You can be walking the hallways or in the tub and be monitored. Be sure to ask what is available at your hospital.

They will also most likely start an IV since it is much easier to get a needle in a laboring woman's vein early in labor than late. This will just be a heparin lock (or hep-lock), the beginnings of an IV, for just-in-case scenarios – just in case you become dehydrated / just in case you ask for pain meds / just in case you need a C-section. It's taped down to your wrist and only attached to an IV pole if needed.

Many families get intimidated in a hospital environment, especially during labor, when they may feel vulnerable and scared. When this happens, it can feel as if others are making decisions about your labor for you, instead of with you. That is not what we want for you! So here is strong acronym I want you to keep at the forefront of your mind as you navigate through decisions regarding your labor and delivery, as well as in to parenting:

B.R.A.I.N.

B – BENEFITS – What are the benefits to our baby and to me?

R – RISKS – What are the risks to our baby and to me?

A – ALTERNATIVES – Are there any alternatives from what you are offering?

I – INTUITION – This is a helpful tool and one not to be ignored. If you need more information, ask for it.

N – NOTHING / NOT NOW – Can we wait a few minutes and try again? Do we *have* to do something?

In many situations during labor, there is time to ask all these questions and make a decision together. By reading this book, you are already empowering yourself with a good amount of knowledge about what to expect, but also about some of the decisions that you may have to make and scenarios that can happen in any labor. All of this can help you stay in control of your labor.

Variance

Internal monitors are occasionally needed in situations where we can't get a good, long read on baby's heartbeat due to position, movement or other factors. Or, if upon listening to baby's heartbeat with the external monitor, your birth team sees potential signs of fetal distress. Internal monitors are basically a magnifying glass on your labor and baby. The illustration below gives you some visual aide in what the tool looks like. A small spiral wire, a scalp electrode, is attached to the top of baby's head – the first layer of skin usually, and this monitors baby's heartbeat. A catheter tube is inserted into the uterus that monitors your contractions in a much more fine-tuned way.

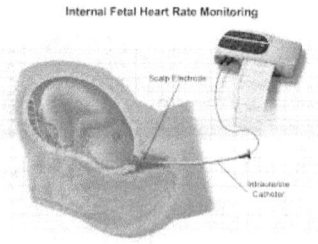

Internal Fetal Heart Rate Monitoring

Let's use B.R.A.I.N. to think about this first possible medical intervention......

Benefits – The benefits are a much clearer picture on how baby is handling labor and contractions

Risks – When the internal monitor is removed from baby's skin, a small droplet (or two) of blood will result, which could also scab for a few days. And if your amniotic sac surrounding baby has not yet broken, they will need to break it in order to get to baby. When this breaks, your risk of infection starts to go up.

Alternatives – If this intervention is being offered because we just can't get a good long read on baby's heartbeat with an external monitor – how about we sit in a warm bath for a bit and see if that relaxes the muscles and helps? Or how about laboring mom walks the hallways for a few minutes and then we try again with the external monitor? If it is being offered because of possible signs of fetal distress, there may not be alternatives.

Intuition – Do you want more information? Does this intervention cause more questions for you? Ask for more information as to why it is needed and wait to decide until you have all the information you need to proceed.

Nothing/not now – Can our laboring mom and her partner or support person have a few minutes to talk it over and decide? Is there an urgency to this or can it wait for a few minutes?

The biggest draw-back with this intervention is the fact that once it is used, it will stay attached to baby until baby is delivered. And what that means for mom is that she will be attached to a machine in the labor and delivery suite, essentially putting her on a 6-foot leash. She will not be able to get in the tub/shower or walk the hallway. Coping techniques can still happen most of the time, but only in your room. The most common time internal monitors are used is when Pitocin is used to induce labor. We will talk more about Pitocin later in this section.

In regards to labor, there a few different pain medications to help a laboring mom if she decides she wants it. They may not all be available at your delivery hospital or through your healthcare provider, so once you read through them, be sure to ask about them at your next appointment to see what options are available for you.

IV NARCOTICS / ANALGESICS – *systemic medication (includes Stadol, Fentanyl, Nubain and Morphine)*

This type of medication is usually described as, "taking the edge off of your contractions." This leads many to believe that means – it helps with the peak of the contraction – the toughest part of it. This is not true. It should instead be described saying that it, "takes the edges off of your contractions." This would better explain that this medication actually makes the ramp up and the ramp down of the contraction a bit fuzzy, tricking your brain into thinking you have more time in between contractions. It does not really touch the peak aspect of contractions. So in turn, it can allow more rest for a laboring mom in between contractions, and for some, this is just what they need to catch their second wind, their sixth wind, their twentieth wind of the day, and come back at it – coping with a peak, then rest, rest, rest, coping with a peak, then rest, rest, rest. For other laboring moms, I describe this as a gateway drug, because they start with IV narcotics, having the edges of their contractions fuzzy, and then they decide that they don't want ANY edges on their contractions – and ask for the next type of pain medication – the Epidural. In most cases, if you start out on IV narcotics and then decide it is not enough, you can still get an epidural. If you started with an epidural, there would not be a need to ask for IV narcotics. Continual monitoring becomes part of your labor any time we are putting something into your body so that we can be sure baby is handling this new element of labor okay, as are you. This means – external monitor belts, a blood pressure cuff taking a reading every 10-20 minutes and an oxygen clip on your finger or toe to be sure your oxygen level in your blood is where it needs to be.

PROS	CONS
Quick to receive / feel relief	Quick to wear off – usually lasts 1.5 hours
-administered by Nurse via shot or IV	
Doesn't affect muscles	Strict cut off of doses long before pushing to ensure out of baby's system
Can allow laboring woman to rest	Nausea possible
	Itchy skin possible
	Trembles possible
	Drop in fetal heart rate possible
	Drop in blood pressure possible
	Can slow labor progress
	Slows production of endorphins so pain may be more intense after drug wears off temporarily

EPIDURAL ANESTHESIA – *Regional anesthetic (such as Bupivacaine, Chloroprocaine, or Lidocaine in combination with opioids or narcotics such as Fentanyl and Sufentanil)*

Epidurals are the most common type of pain medication used in labors across the U.S. They are administered by an Anesthesiologist or a nurse anesthetist at the hospital, usually in your labor and delivery room. Many hospitals have Anesthesiologists dedicated to

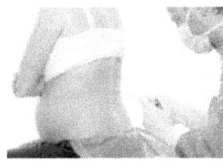
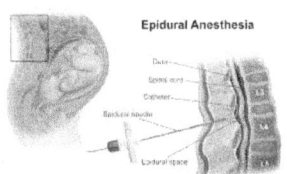

Epidural Anesthesia

labor and delivery, but others do not, and this could be an important factor on your wait time to receive an epidural if you ask

for one and even if you get one. Be sure to ask your healthcare provider about this important detail. The actual procedure to administer the epidural takes about 15 minutes. Pain relief usually begins about 15-30 minutes after administered. Epidurals numb pain sensations in the lower abdomen, back and perineum (area between anus and vagina), allowing a laboring woman to be awake during labor and able to push during delivery – with help. Even with an epidural, it is normal to feel some pressure on the pelvic floor and as baby's head is crowning. Epidurals are preceded by a local anesthetic that numbs the lower back area. This usually causes a stinging sensation in our laboring mom. Once area is numb, an epidural needle is inserted in to the epidural space in her spine and a catheter is threaded through the needle and a small portion is left in the space. The needle is removed and medicine flows to the area through the catheter continuously. The remainder of the catheter is taped to woman's back and mom is guided into a sitting up in bad position while the medicine begins to flow. Sometimes it will begin to make one side of her body more numb than the other and a pillow will be put under one of her hips to help evenly distribute the medication. You will also be given a booster button on a time lock that you can push every once in a while, if you need an additional boost of medicine.

Just like with IV narcotics, continual monitoring of mom and baby will also begin – including a blood pressure cuff taking a reading every 10-20 minutes, external monitor belts, an oxygen clip on your finger or toe to be sure the level of oxygen in your blood is at a safe point, iv fluids through your iv and everyone's favorite – a urinary catheter to empty your bladder.

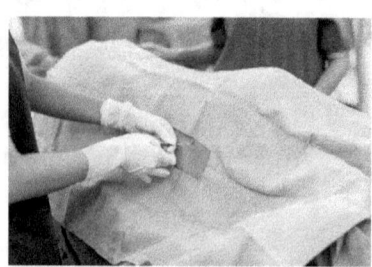

PROS	CONS
Pain relief	Lack of mobility
Allows mom to rest	Lowered fetal heart rate possible
Mental state intact – similar to early labor	Lowered blood pressure possible
Can speed up labor progress	Can slow labor progress
	No food or liquids
	Nausea possible
	Itchy skin possible
	Trembles possible
	Headache possible
	Backache possible
	Bruising at needle insertion sites
	More serious but rare risks are listed on consent form and should be discussed in advance with your healthcare provider

It's good to note that with any hospital intervention, your likelihood of additional interventions increases. One example of this is in regards to some of the cons listed for both of these pain medications – nausea, trembles and itchy skin – there is individual medications to help treat each of those potential side effects – potentially increasing the number of medications you're receiving from 1 to 4.

What about a WALKING EPIDURAL? I've heard about these – can I have one of these instead? – So these, like a mythical unicorn, are a bit misleading in the name. If you have an epidural, you won't be walking anywhere for a while. A walking epidural simply refers to the level of medication you are receiving through the catheter in your spine. It is encouraged to have the level being administered turned as low as you are comfortable for a few reasons, especially as you get close to the pushing stage– 1. Less medication traveling to your baby. 2. More effective pushing because you feel the fuzzy edges of your contractions, as well as have a little less numbing of your legs so you can actually figure out pushing sooner and be better at it. 3. Wears off sooner for you.

NITROUS OXIDE (laughing gas)

This is used frequently in Europe, Canada and Australia but has still not gained wide usage in the U.S. as of this writing. Based on studies I've read and local care givers I've spoken with, the benefits are pretty exciting and the risks minimal. But because it is not widely used as of our publication, I will not include details on it. Do be sure to ask if it available at your hospital and of your healthcare provider. I hope to update this book soon with additional scientific evidence of the pros and cons of this pain medication option, as the usage and studies are increased.

INDUCTION AND AUGMENTATION

INDUCTION

Basically what this means is to use medication or other procedures to start your labor from zero. There needs to be a medical reason to induce your labor. An upcoming holiday or visiting relative is NOT a medical reason to induce. Because there are risks associated with inducing your labor, it is a decision not to be taken lightly. Some of the most common reasons for inductions are:

I.   The amniotic sac has ruptured (water breaks) and contractions don't start on their own in certain amount of time.
II.   Well past your due date – one to two weeks.
III. The health of your baby or your health is at risk.

The two main risks with inducing your labor are:

I.   An increased risk of needing a cesarean delivery
II.   Potential risk of fetal distress

There are a number of methods commonly used to induce labor and it will depend on your individual labor and the factors involved with it, such as baby's health, dilation and cervix ripeness, to name a few.

Let's walk through the variety of options:

Pitocin – The synthetic medication that mimics oxytocin (that our bodies produce naturally) that causes the uterus to contract. It is administered through an IV on a pump system, beginning at a low level and turned up if needed. When a labor is induced with Pitocin, you will often quickly travel through the first stage of labor – Early Labor – and be experiencing Active Labor just a couple hours after beginning your IV. This can be hard on our laboring mom's mental and physical state and she will need support to navigate. This method almost always works to start labor.

Cervical Ripening Medication – Administered in your healthcare provider's office by practioner. Either inserted on or near the cervix or taken orally. Usually a slow release medication used to soften the cervix and get labor started slowly. Multiple doses may be given. Does not always work to get labor started.

Mechanical Dilator – Occasionally used to try to cause the cervix to ripen, using a small bulb device that is inserted in to the cervix and expanded. Has lower risks or fetal distress than other methods but it can increase your risk of infection and require continuous monitoring.

Sweeping the Membranes – Usually done during a vaginal exam at prenatal appointments. Practioner separates the bag of waters from the lower part of the uterus with the hopes that it may cause the release of cervix ripening hormones and eventually cause contractions. There are some recent studies showing that this method may not be as helpful as once thought, and because it is pretty uncomfortable having it done, with potential for bleeding/spotting, along with cramping, be sure your healthcare practioner is asking you if you would like this done and you have all the information you need to make a decision if this is right for you.

So these are all the medical methods used for inducing labor. What are some others that you've heard? Things friends or relatives have tried to get labor started on their own? I know you have some rolling around in your head and some might be great and others can be dangerous. So let's discuss!

First and foremost, all methods to start labor on your own, should be approved and encouraged by your healthcare practioner. This is not something you just want to wing it and stay off of Google! Here are some tried and true methods that potentially can help start labor when you are past your due date and with your practitioner's approval and blessing:

- SEX – So you might say, I'm 42 weeks pregnant, "NO THANKS!" But let me break it down a bit – it is not just the actual act of intercourse that I'm talking about here. In this case, it's all about the orgasm for mom. So get creative – nipple stimulation, massage – think orgasm though. This causes her body to produce oxytocin and remember what that does? It causes the uterus to contract. BINGO! That's what we need. Sperm also carries a natural version of Pitocin, so when it sits on the cervix, it can help it to soften. *So either way -*
- SPICY FOOD – Especially if it is not part of your daily diet, this can, in some cases, get labor started.
- A GREAT PEDICURE – We have a few pressure points on our feet and hands that can send our bodies into labor. And sometimes a strong foot massage can achieve that.
- PREGNANCY MASSAGE – For the same reasons above. If you are getting massages now, your masseuse is avoiding those pressure points, but with your practitioner's permission, they can focus on them and it can be another potential way to get labor started.
- ACCUPUNCTURE/ ACCUPRESSURE – Same reasons listed under pedicure
- BRISK WALK – Sometimes just getting moving can be enough to get labor started.

Your healthcare provider may have other suggestions but best to stay away from herbal remedies, castor oil or any wives' tale suggestions, unless approved by your practitioner, as many can have side effects that can make you miserable and no closer to meeting your baby.

AUGMENTATION

Remember when we talked earlier in the book about how it is very common for labors to stall or stop making progress, most commonly between the 4 – 7 cm dilation stage. When this happens, augmentation is often suggested, which means using medical procedures to restart or improve progress. The two main ways a labor are augmented are using PITOCIN – see description in INDUCTION section, and AROM.

AROM – Artificially rupturing of membranes (or breaking your bag of waters). This is done by your practitioner using a long crochet-type hook with sharp edge. It is inserted into the vaginal canal, feeling like a pelvic exam, where your practioner snags the sac and pulls back, causing it to rupture. This can only be done when baby's head is low enough in the birth canal so to reduce any risk of cord prolapse (See C-Section section). Once ruptured, it causes baby's head to drop against the cervix, hoping the increase in pressure will cause the contraction strength to increase.

SECOND STAGE INTERVENTIONS

Occasionally, an intervention is needed to assist your baby through the birth canal during pushing and these are referred to as second stage interventions. The two main reasons they could be needed are:

I.   Signs of fetal distress

II.   Pushing is made difficult due to exhaustion, pain medication, baby size or position

There are two main interventions used-

VACUUM EXTRACTOR – A small and flexible cup connected with a tube to a vacuum source, often a hand pump. The pump will create a suction hold on the top of baby's head and over the course of usually just 3 contractions, while mom is push, push, pushing – your practitioner will be gently pulling on baby.

Vacuum-assisted Delivery

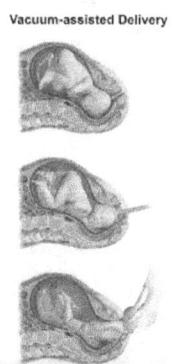

Using a vacuum extractor for only approximately 3 contractions is pretty standard for two reasons – the main one being that babies are not big fans of this and can show signs of fetal distress. And the other reason being that if progress is not made over 3 contractions, it most likely won't be made, and baby needs to be delivered via unplanned C-section. There are many successful vacuum extracted births though and it is widely used by both Midwives and OBGYNs.

FORCEPS – Metal spoon-like instruments that fit around either side of baby's head and just like with the vacuum extractor, they

can be tried over approximately 3 contractions – mom is push, push, pushing and practitioner is gently pulling.

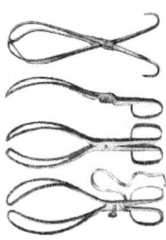

Forceps are less common than the vacuum extractor, many OBGYNs do use them on a regular basis as needed. Having options to assist baby's delivery can help avoid an unnecessary C-section, but it is also important to note there are risks involved with the mentioned interventions.

The potential risks are:

- Bruising or bumps on the baby's head
- Tearing of the perineum, vagina or anus
- Nerve problems (temporary) in baby's face (forceps)

A cesarean birth can best be described as the surgical delivery of your baby via an incision in a mother's belly and then uterus. C-section rates, although on the decline, are hovering at about 32% of all labors across the U.S., as of data from 2015. There are different types of C-sections and different reasons they might be needed.

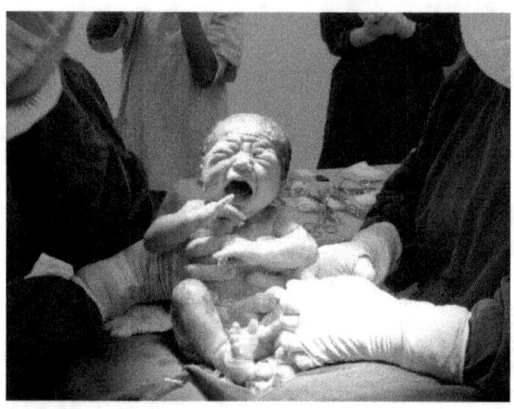

PLANNED C-Sections

As their name suggests, these deliveries are planned in advance, usually close to your due date and should not be done for elective reasons, only when medically needed. Some reasons for a planned C-section would be:

- Baby's position – usually Breech – when baby bottom or feet are near the opening of the uterus instead of the head. Or Transverse – baby is turned sideways in uterus.
- Previous C-section delivery – if mom is not a contender for a VBAC (Vaginal delivery after C-section) – a planned C-Section might be only delivery option.
- Twins or multiples – twins are more likely to at least be allowed to try for a vaginal delivery but not multiples.
- Placenta Previa – placenta is blocking the cervix.
- Medical problems – you or baby – that may have been pre-existing or materialize during or due to pregnancy.

UNPLANNED C-Sections

The need for a C-section occasionally arise during labor, again not for convenience but when a medical need drives the decision. Some reasons that could arise that could lead to an unplanned C-section are:

- Abnormal fetal heart rate – fetal distress not improving by external methods
- Meconium present in amniotic fluid – meaning that baby had their first bowel movement in utero and that waste is now being inhaled and digested by baby. If not at pushing stage, this can be a reason for an unplanned C-section.
- Labor not progressing despite all possible augmentation methods
- Baby's position – during labor, baby moves in to a non-ideal delivery position (breech or transverse)
- CPD (Cephalopelvic disproportion), basically meaning that baby's head does not fit through the pelvis.

With both PLANNED and UNPLANNED C-Sections, the mother is awake and alert throughout the procedure. She does not feel pain but she does often feel tugging and pushing as baby is delivered. Most hospitals will allow at least one support person in to the OR for a C-section. Some will also allow a Doula or second support person in as well. Be sure to check on the policy with your healthcare provider. Support person will need to put scrubs over clothing, shoes and hair before the surgery because the OR is a sterile environment. The best place for your partner or support person during the entire surgery, is seated in the chair by the head of the bed. This is important for a few reasons – 1. Even if they can handle the most gruesome movie ever, watching this surgery on their beloved is not the same. And if they pass out in the OR, there are no second chances. They will be taken to a recovery room and left there to wait for the surgery to be over and mom and baby to join them in the recovery room. If they are really curious, they can ask questions in the OR and to know what is happening, or even watch it on someone else on YouTube well after your baby is born and home. 2. The second and even more important reason for them to be stationed in the chair by mom's head is this – many moms are not planning on delivering via C-section and will be going through a very tough emotional journey during the procedure. They will need their partner's love and support and reassurance that this is the best way for mom and baby to cross that finish line – healthy and safe.

Planned and unplanned C-sections usually take about an hour to perform, with baby being born just about 20 minutes in to that hour. If you have a Midwife, the on call OB will perform the surgery and your Midwife will assist in the OR. The doctor makes a 4-6-inch incision (horizontal) just above the pubic hairline, in the skin and fatty tissue. Then the abdominal muscles are separated and retracted to expose the uterus. The doctor makes another incision in to the uterus and gently guides baby away from the birth canal and out of the incision opening, while an assistant press on the top of the uterus. Upon baby's birth, that is usually when you can take the first amazing photos. Some hospitals are allowing partner or support people to cut the umbilical cord if the situation allows it, but you will have to check on that policy at your delivery hospital. Many hospitals are also initiating skin-to-skin right after delivery now too, which aides in baby's transition, breathing, temperature, blood sugar and heart rate, along with mom's healing. Here too though, every hospital has different policies, so be sure to ask your healthcare provider what to expect at yours if a C-section becomes part of your birth.

Once baby is born, the delivery team delivers the placenta and repairs the incision sites. After the surgery is complete, mom and baby are taken to a recovery room, where after newborn procedures are completed, they will learn how to breastfeed. You can usually plan on being in the hospital approximately 56 - 72 hours after delivery if baby was delivered via C-section.

EMERGENCY C-Section

The last type of C-section is rare and only equates for about 1% of all births every year in the U.S. During an emergency C-section, mom is usually given general anesthesia so they can put her to sleep and work quickly. This is also the only type of C-section that a partner or support person is not able to attend. The main reasons for an emergency C-section are:

- Cord prolapse – Where the umbilical cord precedes baby through the cervix and as baby descends, it can pinch the cord, cutting off the oxygen flow to baby.
- Placenta abruption – the placenta detaches from the uterine wall before baby is born, causing severe bleeding.
- Uterine rupture – a tear in the uterine wall that can cause severe bleeding and fetal distress.

So although a C-section is a possibility in any birth, it is **not** a probability in most births.

Some preventive things you can do to reduce your risks of a C-sections delivery are:

- Stay at home in early labor to increase the likelihood of labor continuing to progress and not stall
- Wait as long as you can in labor, if you opt for an epidural, to avoid the medication slowing or stopping your labor
- Avoid induction as a convenience and only use if it becomes medically necessary
- Try to stay within the weight gain limits set by your healthcare provider during pregnancy
- Change positions frequently – using gravity and movement to help baby down and out of the birth canal
- Have a good support system leading up to and during labor

You made it through labor and delivery and all the avenues of possibility between. You hopefully now have plenty of information to do this yourself and feel empowered doing it! You are just about to start one of the best journeys of your life as a mom and I hope you feel more ready. Don't be afraid to be your own advocate and ask questions and ask for support. Whatever path your birth takes, it is only **YOUR** business and no one else's. Try to shield yourself from other's opinions, because it's not their birth – it's yours. *However,* you get across that finish line – I wish for you a healthy baby, healthy mom and a deep, deep positive perspective on your special day!

Congratulations and thanks for reading my book!

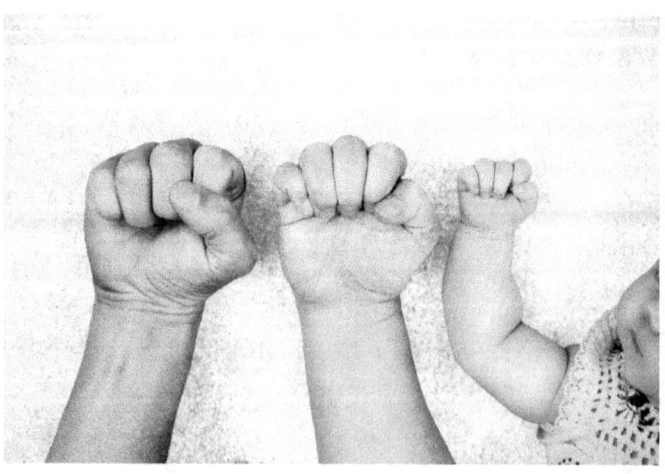

A special thank you to my family for always supporting me in everything I do – my children, Taylor, Morgan, Jack and Nate - You guys are my heart.

Thank you also to:

Swedish Hospital Seattle

IStock / Adobe Stock

Wikipedia

TeamMommy

The Seattle Doula Community

Seattle Midwifery (Now Bastyr University)

Great Starts

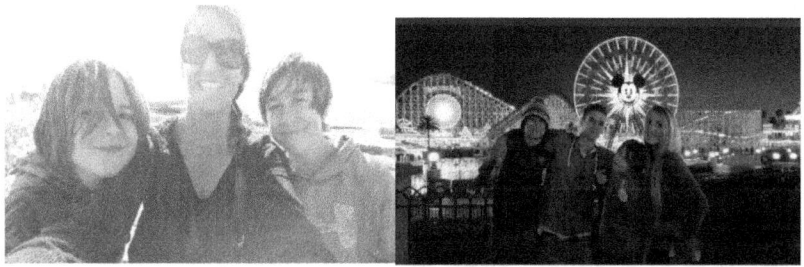

Western Washington University

Wishing you wonderful adventures ahead as a parent –

from my family to yours!

*Keep an eye out for additional books being released soon:

Postpartum Recovery and a Plan

Newborn Care – from Breastfeeding to Tummy Time